I0704315

Prostate Cancer Survival:

A simple and effective guide to overcome the odds and reclaim your life

By

Dr. Edward A. Johnson

Copyright © by Dr. Edward A. Johnson 2023.
All rights reserved.
Before this document is duplicated or reproduced in any manner, the publisher's consent must be gained. Therefore, the contents within can neither be stored electronically, transferred, nor kept in a database.
Neither in part nor full can the document be copied, scanned, faxed or retained without approval from the publisher or creator.

1

Table of contents

Introduction
Prostate cancer: what is it?
Why does prostate cancer develop?
Types of prostate cancer
Symptoms and Causes
What are the prostate cancer risk factors?
TESTS AND DIAGNOSIS
methods for diagnosing prostate cancer
CONTROL AND TREATMENT
Prevention
PROGNOSIS
LIVING WITH PROSTATE CANCER
Metastatic prostate cancer
Treatment
Maintaining a Healthful Lifestyle
Age, race, and genes are factors you cannot change.
Diet and lifestyle changes are things you can make.
Natural Methods for Preventing Prostate Cancer
What to Avoid
Other Ways to Avoid Prostate Cancer
Conclusion

Introduction

Prostate cancer is the most frequently diagnosed male cancer and the fifth most prevalent cause of cancer mortality in males worldwide. Globally, this sickness caused 1,414,249 newly diagnosed cases and 375,000 fatalities in 2020. Prostate cancer is the most prevalent malignancy detected globally in more than 50% of countries (112 of 185).

Thankfully, the majority of prostate tumors grow slowly, are low-grade, have a modest risk, and are not particularly aggressive.

In the majority of instances, there are no initial or early symptoms, but late symptoms can include anemia-related weariness, bone pain, spinal metastases-related paralysis, and renal failure from bilateral ureteral obstruction. Prostate-specific antigen (PSA) testing and transrectal ultrasound-guided (TRUS) prostate tissue biopsies are the mainstays of diagnosis, while PSA testing for screening is still debatable.

Free and total PSA levels, PCA3 urine testing, PHI, the "4K" test, exosome testing, genomic analysis, MRI imaging, PIRADS scoring, and MRI-TRUS fusion-guided biopsies are examples of more recent diagnostic techniques.

Prostate-specific cancer is regarded as confined and potentially treatable when it only affects the prostate.

Painkillers, bisphosphonates, rank ligand inhibitors, hormone therapy, chemotherapy, radiopharmaceuticals, immunotherapy, focused radiation, and other targeted therapies may be utilized if the illness has progressed to the bones or locations other than the prostate. Age, accompanying health issues, tumor histology, and the degree of malignancy all affect outcomes.

Prostate cancer: what is it?

Cancer is a condition in which the body's cells proliferate unchecked. The prostate's cells are where prostate cancer first develops. A gland in the male reproductive system is the prostate. It is situated close to the bladder. Fluid, a component of semen, is produced.

Prostate cancer is one of the most common cancers. It frequently progresses very slowly. It might not pose a major threat if it does not spread to other bodily regions. Yet, prostate cancer can occasionally develop swiftly and disperse to other bodily regions. Prostate cancer of this type is dangerous.

Although it is a frequent kind of cancer in men, prostate cancer is very treatable in its early stages. It begins in the prostate gland, which is situated between the penis and the bladder. Although the cause is unknown to experts, the danger rises with age.

The prostate serves several purposes. They include releasing PSA, a protein that helps semen maintain its liquid state, generating the fluid that nourishes and transports sperm, and assisting with urinary control.

Prostate cancer is the most prevalent cancer afflicting men in the US, other than skin cancer. According to the American Cancer Society (ACS), there will be roughly 34,130 prostate cancer fatalities and 248,530 new cases of prostate cancer in 2021.

Prostate cancer will be diagnosed in about 1 in 8 men at some time in their lives. Yet, just 1 in 41 will die as a result. This is due to early-stage cancers having efficient treatments and later-stage cancers having slow-growing characteristics. The majority of prostate cancer cases can be found by doctors through routine screening before they spread.

Why does prostate cancer develop?

Prostate cancer's exact cause is unknown to researchers. They are aware that it occurs when the genetic material is altered (DNA).

You are born with these genetic changes if they are inherited on occasion. Additionally, some genetic changes can raise your lifelong risk of developing prostate cancer. Yet, the particular cause of these genetic changes is typically unknown.

In men and those born with masculine gender identity, the prostate, a small walnut-shaped gland situated behind the bladder and in front of the rectum, develops into prostate cancer (AMAB). This small gland produces fluid that mixes with semen to preserve the health of the sperm for pregnancy and fertilization.

The disease of prostate cancer is dangerous. Thankfully, the majority of men with prostate cancer are identified before the disease has spread past the prostate gland. When cancer is treated at this stage, it frequently vanishes.

Types of prostate cancer

Adenocarcinoma is most likely the type of prostate cancer you have if you are diagnosed with it. Adenocarcinomas begin in the cells of glands that release fluid, such as your prostate. Rarely, different cell types can develop into prostate cancer.
The following prostate cancer subtypes are less frequent:
• Small cell carcinomas.
• Cancers of the transitional cells.
neuroendocrine tumors.
• Sarcomas.

How common is Prostate cancer?

As the most frequent disease affecting men and individuals AMAB, prostate cancer is relatively common, coming in second only to skin cancer. 13 men with prostates out of every 100 will eventually get prostate cancer, according to the U.S. Centers for Disease Control and Prevention (CDC). Most men will lead regular lives and pass away from diseases unrelated to prostate cancer in the end. Some patients won't require care.

Nonetheless, every year, 34,000 Americans lose their lives to prostate cancer.

Who has a higher risk of developing prostate cancer?

Prostate cancer can strike everyone who has one. Yet, some things can increase your risk of getting it:

• **Age.** As you age, your risk of having prostate cancer rises. In men under the age of 50, prostate cancer is uncommon.

• **A family's medical history.** If either of your parents, a sibling, or a kid has or had prostate cancer, your risk of developing the disease is increased.

• **Race.** African Americans are more likely to develop prostate cancer. Also, they are more likely to develop prostate cancer earlier in life and with more advanced diseases.

• Perish due to prostate cancer.

Prostate cancer will be discovered in about 1 in 7 men at some point in their lives. Moreover, research suggests that a large number of elderly men have undetected prostate cancer, which is not aggressive, unlikely to present symptoms, and unlikely to shorten their lifetime. Prostate cancer is the second most prevalent cause of cancer death among males in the United States, even though the majority of men who are diagnosed with it do not pass away from it. Prostate cancer is uncommon before the age of 40, and more than 60% of cases are discovered beyond age 65. Black Americans in the United States are more likely than males of other ethnic origins to get prostate cancer, and they are also more likely to die from the condition.

Symptoms and Causes

Which signs and symptoms accompany prostate cancer?

Rarely do symptoms of early-stage prostate cancer appear. As the illness advances, several problems could arise:
• Often needing to urinate urgently, especially at night.
• Weak urine flow or intermittent urine flow.
• Burning or aching when urinating (dysuria).
• A decline in bladder control (urinary incontinence).
• Abnormal bowel movements (fecal incontinence).
• Erectile dysfunction and painful ejaculation (ED).
• Hematospermia, or blood in the sperm or urine.
• Chest, hip, or low back pain.

Advanced signs

Advanced prostate cancer patients may also go undiagnosed. Cancer's size and the extent of its internal dissemination will determine any potential symptoms. The following signs and symptoms of advanced prostate cancer can also be present:
• unexpected weight loss and bone pain
• tiredness

Are issues with the prostate necessarily indicative of prostate cancer?

Not all prostate growths are cancerous. Other ailments that manifest prostate cancer-like symptoms include:
• **Benign prostatic hyperplasia (BPH):** This condition affects nearly everyone who has a prostate at some point (BPH). This condition enlarges your prostate gland without raising your risk of developing cancer.
• **Prostatitis:** If you're under 50, an enlarged prostate gland most certainly signifies the

condition if it's present. Your prostate gland might become inflamed and swollen due to the benign illness known as prostatitis. Infections with bacteria are frequently to blame.

What causes prostate cancer?

What makes cells in your prostate develop into cancer cells is unknown to experts. Prostate cancer develops when cells divide more quickly than usual, just like other cancers do. Cancer cells do not eventually die, but normal cells do. Instead, they proliferate and develop into a lump known as a tumor. Parts of the tumor may separate and spread to other areas of your body as the cells continue to divide (metastasize). Fortunately, prostate cancer typically advances slowly. The majority of tumors are discovered before your prostate has been affected by the disease. At this point, prostate cancer is quite curable.

What are the prostate cancer risk factors?

The most typical risk elements are:

• **Age.** Becoming older puts you at greater risk. If you're over 50, you have a higher chance of being diagnosed. Prostate cancer affects adults older than 65 in about 60% of cases.

• **Ethnicity and race.** If you are Black or have African ancestry, you are at higher risk. You have a higher chance of developing prostate tumors that spread quickly. Moreover, you have a higher chance of developing prostate cancer before age 50.

• **History of prostate cancer in the family.** If you have a close relative who has prostate cancer, your risk of developing it is two to three times higher.

• **Genetics.** If you have Lynch syndrome or inherited altered (mutated) genes linked to an

elevated chance of developing breast cancer, your risk is higher (BRCA1 and BRCA2).
• **Diet:** According to some data, eating a lot of fat may make you more likely to get prostate cancer.
Several prostate cancer risk factors have been discovered in certain studies, however, the evidence is conflicting. Smoking is one more risk factor that could be present.
• Prostatitis.
• A BMI of 30 or above (having obesity).
Sexually transmitted diseases (STIs).
• Contact with Agent Orange (a chemical used during the Vietnam War)

TESTS AND DIAGNOSIS

Exactly how is prostate cancer identified?

Prostate cancer can be early detected thanks to screenings. By age 55, if your risk is average, you'll likely get your first screening procedure. If you belong to a high-risk category, you could require earlier testing. Screenings typically come to an end at age 70.

If screenings reveal that you may have prostate cancer, you may need additional testing or procedures.

Testing for prostate cancer detection

If you need further testing due to prostate cancer symptoms, screening tests can reveal this.

• **Digital rectal examination:** When you receive a (DRE), the doctor inserts a gloved, lubricated finger into your rectum to feel for any prostate lumps, rigidity, or enlargement.

This approach may be used to detect prostate cancer because it frequently begins at the back of the gland. It is more beneficial in men who still have prostate cancer while having an average PSA level, even if it is not as effective as a PSA test.

• **Blood test for prostate-specific antigen (PSA):** Protein-specific antigen is a protein that the prostate gland produces (PSA). Elevated PSA levels could be a sign of cancer. Moreover, levels increase if you have benign diseases like BPH or prostatitis.

Both healthy and malignant prostate cells produce the protein known as PSA or prostate-specific antigen. All males typically have some PSA in their blood.

A high PSA score may indicate malignancy. But, prostate diseases that are not cancerous might also cause your PSA level to increase. For instance, if you have an infection of the urine.

A PSA level alone cannot be used to diagnose prostate cancer.

Talking about the test

The potential drawbacks and advantages of a PSA test should be discussed with your doctor. The PSA level is not a good indicator of a man's prostatic cancer status. Although some men have prostate cancer, their PSA levels are within the usual range for their age. Some men, who do not have prostate cancer, have higher PSA levels. Also, a PSA test is only worthwhile if you are healthy enough to receive treatment if you are found to have prostate cancer.

Your doctor ought to go over the test with you and allow you adequate time to talk to your spouse or other members of your family about it.

Interpreting the results of your PSA test

The standard unit of measurement for PSA is nanograms per milliliter of blood (ng/ml). There isn't a single PSA value that is regarded as normal. As you age, the reading changes from man to man and the level rises. The average PSA level in men is less than 3ng/ml.

If your PSA level is higher than what is considered typical for your age, your doctor could recommend that you see a specialist. It's critical to keep in mind that elderly men may have normal PSA levels beyond 3ng/ml. Discuss your PSA level and what it implies for you with your doctor.

In most cases, doctors abide by recommendations that specify when to send a patient to a specialist. The various UK countries have slightly varying versions of these rules. It's crucial to understand that your doctor decides who needs to see a specialist based on their knowledge and discretion.

If your PSA level is: your doctor may recommend that you see a specialist.

Age	PSA score
40 to 49	greater than 2.5ng/ml
50 to 59	more than 3.5ng/ml
60 to 69	more than 4.5ng/ml
70 to 79	more than 6.5ng/ml

If you are younger than 40 or older than 79, your doctor will exercise their discretion.

If you are sent to a specialist, they will examine you physically and look for any additional symptoms you may be experiencing. After that, you might undergo additional testing including an MRI scan and a biopsy.

What influences the level of PSA?

Other than cancer, various conditions might cause the PSA level to vary.

Before doing a test, your doctor may want to rule out a urinary infection. You should wait at least 6 weeks before getting a PSA test if you recently had a urinary infection.

Additional elements that influence your PSA level are:

• ejaculation within the previous 48 hours; a prostate exam (digital rectal examination) performed before the PSA blood test; strenuous activity within the previous 48 hours; and a prostate biopsy performed within the previous six weeks.

There are many recommendations for how much time should pass between engaging in these activities and taking a PSA test. Find out from your doctor what they advise.

PSA for "Free and Bound"

There are various PSA forms. It may be either free (not connected to proteins) or bound (associated with other blood proteins).

The amount of free and bound PSA in the blood is determined by the routine PSA test.

Prostate cancer screening

The UK does not have a nationwide prostate cancer screening program. This is due to earlier studies demonstrating that the PSA test is unreliable for detecting prostate cancer that requires therapy. A new test is being looked for through research. Or to determine if the current test might be more successful if applied differently.

Ask your doctor whether you want a PSA test if you are over 50. Your doctor can go over the potential dangers of having this test with you. They will assist you in deciding whether or not to take the test.

methods for diagnosing prostate cancer

Not every person with prostate cancer will require a certain diagnosis. For instance, if your doctor believes that your tumor is developing slowly, they can decide against conducting any additional testing since they don't think it has to be treated. You could require more tests, such as a biopsy if it's more aggressive (growing quickly or spreading).

Not every person with prostate cancer will require a certain diagnosis. For instance, if your tumor is believed to be slow-growing, your doctor may decide to postpone additional testing because it isn't seen to be significant enough to warrant treatment. You could require more tests, such as a biopsy if it's more aggressive (growing quickly or spreading).

• **Imaging:** Your prostate gland can be seen on a transrectal ultrasound or an MRI, including any abnormal regions that might be cancer. Imaging data can assist your doctor in determining whether to take a biopsy or not.

• **Biopsy:** During a needle biopsy, a medical professional takes a sample of tissue to be examined for malignancy in a lab. The only reliable approach to identify prostate cancer or determine its aggressiveness is through a biopsy. The biopsy tissue may be subjected to genetic testing by your doctor. Certain cancer cells contain traits (such as mutations) that increase their propensity to respond to particular therapies.

What prostate cancer classifications and stages are there?

To establish the severity of the disease and the kinds of therapies you require, healthcare professionals use the Gleason score and cancer staging.

Gleason rating

Your doctor can evaluate how abnormal your cancer cells are using the Gleason score. Your Gleason score increases as the number of aberrant cells increases. Your doctor can assess your cancer's grade or potential for aggression using the Gleason score.

prostate cancer staging

Your doctor can assess the stage of your cancer and how far it has spread by doing so. Your prostate gland may simply have localized (local) cancer, or it may have regional (regional) cancer or have spread to other organs (metastasized). Your lymph nodes and bones are the most typical sites where prostate cancer spreads. Other organs such as the liver, brain, lungs, and others may also develop it.

CONTROL AND TREATMENT

How are these conditions managed or treated?

Your overall health, whether cancer has spread, and how quickly it is spreading are just a few of the variables that will affect how you will be treated. You might collaborate with urologists, radiation oncologists, and medical oncologists depending on your therapy options. Most prostate cancers that are discovered in their early stages can be treated and recovered from.

specific methods employed

Surveillance

If your cancer grows slowly and doesn't spread, your doctor may choose to monitor your situation rather than treat you.

• **Active surveillance:** To track the progression of cancer, you undergo screenings, scans, and biopsies every one to three years. If the cancer is only in your prostate, is growing slowly, and

isn't causing any symptoms, active surveillance is the most effective. Your doctor can begin treating you if your problem gets worse.

• **Watchful waiting:** Similar to active monitoring, watchful waiting is more frequently employed for frailer cancer patients whose condition is unlikely to improve with treatment. Testing occurs significantly less frequently as well. Treatments frequently concentrate on treating symptoms rather than removing the tumor.

Surgery

A damaged prostate gland is removed during radical prostatectomy. It frequently eradicates prostate tumors that haven't progressed. If your doctor thinks you would benefit from this procedure, they can advise you on the optimal removal technique.

• **Open radical prostatectomy:** Your doctor removes your prostate gland by a single abdominal incision that extends from your belly button to your pubic bone. Compared to less

invasive procedures like robotic prostatectomy, this technique is less common.

• **Robotic radical prostatectomy:** With this procedure, your surgeon can operate through some small incisions. They use a console to control a robot system rather than directly controlling it.

radiation treatment

Radiation therapy can be used alone or in conjunction with other therapies to treat prostate cancer. Furthermore, radiation may help with symptoms.

• **Brachytherapy:** This internal radiation therapy entails implanting radioactive seeds inside your prostate. With this method, cancer cells are destroyed but surrounding healthy tissue is kept intact.

• **External beam radiation therapy (EBRT):** This procedure uses a machine to direct potent

27

X-ray beams at the tumor. High doses of radiation can be directed at the tumor while still protecting

healthy tissue with specialized EBRT techniques like IMRT.

Integrated treatments

If cancer has gone beyond your prostate gland, your doctor might advise systemic therapy. Systemic therapy circulates drugs throughout your body to kill cancer cells or stop them from proliferating.

• **Hormone treatment:** Testosterone promotes the proliferation of cancer cells. To counter testosterone's contribution to the proliferation of cancer cells, hormone treatment employs medicines. The drugs either lower your testosterone levels or stop testosterone from getting to cancer cells, which is how they function. As an alternative, your doctor can advise having your testicles surgically removed (orchiectomy) to stop them from producing testosterone. Those who prefer not to use medicine can choose this operation.

• **Chemotherapy:** This treatment employs drugs to kill cancer cells. If your cancer has gone past your prostate, you may undergo hormone

treatment in addition to or instead of chemotherapy.

• **Immunotherapy:** Immunotherapy fortifies your immune system, enhancing its capacity to recognize and combat cancer cells. Immunotherapy may be suggested by your doctor to treat advanced cancer or recurrent cancer (cancer that goes away but then returns).

• **Targeted therapy:** To stop cancer cells from proliferating and reproducing, targeted therapy focuses on the genetic alterations (mutations) that transform healthy cells into cancer cells. Cancer cells with BRCA gene abnormalities are destroyed by targeted therapy for prostate cancer.

Targeted treatment

A more recent method of treatment called focal therapy eliminates malignancies inside the prostate. If the cancer is low risk and hasn't spread, your doctor might advise this treatment. The majority of these therapies are currently regarded as experimental.

• **High-intensity focused ultrasound (HIFU):** Strong heat is produced by high-intensity sound waves to eliminate cancer cells in your prostate.
• Cryotherapy: Cold gases freeze prostate cancer cells, removing the tumor.
• **Laser ablation:** By killing the cancer cells in your prostate with intense heat, the tumor is removed.
• **Drugs increase the sensitivity of cancer cells** to specific light wavelengths. These light wavelengths are applied by a medical professional to eliminate cancer cells.

What potentially harmful effects could prostate cancer treatment have?

Possible negative effects include:

• **Incontinence:** Even when your bladder isn't full, you could leak urine when you cough, laugh or have an intense urge to urinate. Without treatment, this issue often gets better throughout the first six to twelve months.

• **Erectile dysfunction (ED):** Surgery, radiation, and other medical procedures might harm your penis' erectile nerves, which can impair your capacity to achieve or sustain an erection. Within a year or two, it's typical to regain erectile function (sometimes sooner). Drugs like sildenafil (Viagra) or tadalafil (Cialis) can aid in the interim by boosting blood flow to your penis.

• **Infertility:** Medical procedures may impair your capacity to create or ejaculate sperm, which might lead to infertility. Before beginning therapy, you can store sperm in a sperm bank if you intend to have children in the future. After therapy, you might have sperm extracted. With this process, sperm is directly removed from testicular tissue and implanted into the uterus of your spouse.

If you are having any side effects from your treatment, consult your doctor. They frequently have helpful recommendations for medications and treatments.

Prevention

How can I avoid developing prostate cancer?

Prostate cancer cannot be prevented. Even so, following these instructions may lower your risk:

• **Have regular prostate exams.** According to your risk factors, ask your healthcare professional how frequently you should get checked.

• **Continue to be a healthy weight.** Find out from your doctor what a healthy weight is for you.

• **Regular exercise.** More than 20 minutes of moderate-intensity activity each day, or 150 minutes per week, is advised by the CDC.

• **Have a balanced diet.** While there isn't a single diet that will prevent cancer, healthy eating practices can enhance your general well-being. eat entire grains, fruits, and veggies. Steer clear of processed foods and red meat.

• **Give up smoking.** Don't use tobacco products. If you smoke, work on quitting with the help of your healthcare physician.

PROGNOSIS

How likely is it that someone with prostate cancer will survive?

If your healthcare professional finds prostate cancer early, your prognosis is great. 99% of people who are diagnosed with prostate cancer that hasn't gone elsewhere survive for at least five years after their diagnosis.

When the disease has metastasized or spread outside of your prostate, your chances of surviving prostate cancer are less favorable. Five years later, 32 percent of men with metastatic prostate cancer are still alive.

How treatable is prostate cancer?

Certainly, if it's discovered quickly. In certain instances, cancer grows so slowly that immediate therapy may not be necessary. Prostate tumors that have not progressed past the prostate gland are frequently curable.

LIVING WITH PROSTATE CANCER

When should I make a call to my doctor?

• Trouble urinating is a sign that you need to see your healthcare practitioner.

• Often peeing (incontinence).
• Pain during urination or sexual contact.
• Blood in your urination or sperm.

What inquiries should I make to my doctor?

Ask your doctor the following questions if you have prostate cancer:

• Has my prostate gland's cancer spread to other organs?
• Which course of action is recommended for my stage of prostate cancer?
• What are the dangers and side effects of the medication?
• Does my family have a high chance of prostate cancer? Should we undergo genetic testing if so?
• What sort of post-treatment care do I require? Should I be on the lookout for complications?

Survival of prostate cancer

Many variables are necessary for survival.
Nobody can predict your exact life expectancy.
The general figures shown here are based on
sizable populations. Remember that they cannot
foretell how your specific case would turn out.

In general, prostate cancer survivors have an
excellent prognosis, especially if they receive an
early diagnosis.

Continuity by stage

Statistics on prostate cancer survival by stage are
not available for the entire United Kingdom.
For every stage of prostate cancer, survival data
are available in England. For those who were
diagnosed between 2013 and 2017, these
statistics apply.

Stage 1:
Stage 1 refers to prostate cancer that has spread
to less than half of one side of the prostate.
Within the prostate gland, it is entirely enclosed.

Nearly everyone (nearly 100%) will remain cancer-free for at least five years after being diagnosed.

Stage 2:

Stage 2 signifies that prostate cancer has spread to more than half of one side. But the prostate gland is still totally able to contain it.

Nearly everyone (nearly 100%) will remain cancer-free for at least five years after being diagnosed.

Stage 3:

Stage 3 signifies that the prostate gland's covering (capsule) has been compromised by the malignancy. It might have entered sperm transport tubes (seminal vesicles).

95 out of 100 males (or about 95%) will remain cancer-free for at least five years after being diagnosed.

Stage 4:

Stage 4 can refer to a variety of things, such as:

• cancer has spread to surrounding lymph nodes;
• cancer has spread to body parts outside of the pelvis, such as the lungs or liver; cancer has spread into nearby body organs, such as the bladder or the back passage;
50% of males will remain cancer-free for at least five years after being diagnosed, or about 50 out of 100 men.

Survival rates for prostate cancer at all stages

Typically for English males with prostate cancer:

• More than 95 percent of those with cancer will live with it for a year or longer.
• More than 85 out of 100 (more than 85%) people with cancer will live for at least 5 years after diagnosis.
• Almost 80% of people with cancer will live for at least 10 years after being diagnosed.
Scotland and Northern Ireland have both documented prostate cancer survivorship.

However, due to variations in the methods used to get the data, comparing survival rates between these nations is challenging.

Determinants of survival

Depending on cancer's stage at the time of diagnosis, your prognosis will change. This refers to the size of the problem and its spread. Your chance of survival is also influenced by the grade and type of prostate cancer. Using a microscope, grade refers to how aberrant the

cells appear. The Gleason score is the most widely used criterion for classifying prostate cancer. A higher Gleason score indicates a worse future for men.

Your PSA level affects your outlook as well. Your cancer may spread more quickly if your PSA level is high.

Your general fitness and health have an impact on survival. Your ability to deal with your cancer and therapy will improve as your fitness level increases.

Metastatic prostate cancer

Prostate cancer that has spread to other body organs is referred to as metastatic prostate cancer. It is referred to as advanced prostate cancer occasionally. The bones or lymph nodes in other places of the body are where it spreads most frequently. Moreover, other organs may become affected.

Aggressive prostate cancer locally

Prostate cancer that has spread locally differs from prostate cancer that has progressed.

Locally progressed prostate cancer refers to the disease's invasion of lymph nodes and surrounding tissue. The tissue surrounding the prostate and the tubes that deliver sperm are two areas where it might have spread. They include the seminal vesicles, surrounding bodily structures like the bladder or the back channel, and lymph nodes close to the prostate gland.

What regions spread prostate cancer?

Although prostate cancer can spread to any organ, it most frequently travels to the following:
• bones
• lymph nodes
• live
• lungs.
If you experience any symptoms that could be related to metastatic prostate cancer, your doctor will schedule several scans and tests. Also, they

will examine you and ask you how you are
feeling.

TNM phases

Tumor, Node, and Metastasis is the abbreviation
for the TNM staging system.

Both T and N provide information on the tumor's
size and the presence of cancerous cells in the
lymph nodes, respectively.

According to the TNM staging method,
metastatic prostate cancer is classified as any T,

any N, or M1. M1 indicates if cancer has
migrated to another area of the body.

Tests to identify prostate cancer that has spread

Tests to identify metastatic prostate cancer may
be performed on you. You may have undergone
some of these tests in the past since they can be
comparable to those used to diagnose prostate
cancer.

Treatment

Your response to treatment will depend on

• your age

• your general health

• how you feel about the side effects and therapies.

Several therapies are available for metastatic prostate cancer. They consist of:

• chemotherapy

• radiation

• steroids

• hormone treatment

• targeted medications

• Radioisotope therapy

• symptom management, such as therapy for bone pain

Perhaps feeling

Prostate cancer cannot be cured after it has progressed. But, medication can keep it under control for a while and aid with symptom relief. It is upsetting and can come as a shock to learn that your cancer cannot be treated. It's normal to feel uneasy and uncertain. It's common to have nothing else on your mind.

You, your family, and your friends have access to a wealth of knowledge and assistance. Learning more about your cancer and any potential treatments can be beneficial. Many people discover that being more informed about their circumstances can help them cope.

Speak with your doctor or nurse to learn more about your diagnosis, what is likely to happen, the treatments available to you, and how they can help you.

A group of medical experts who can help you will take care of you and your family.

Survival

Many people are interested in the prognosis and course of their cancer. Each person will experience this differently. All the details concerning you and your cancer are in the hands of your cancer specialist. The best person to talk to about this is them.

Maintaining a Healthful Lifestyle

There is no one strategy to prevent prostate cancer, even though many people may question how to do so. Maintaining good health as you age or taking action to address any health issues can reduce your risk. However, just like all malignancies, some risk factors for prostate cancer must be prevented.

Age, race, and genes are factors you cannot change.

Mostly an "aging disease," prostate cancer. The likelihood of having prostate cancer rises with age. Race and heredity also play a significant role. In comparison to white American males, African American men have twice as high a risk of acquiring prostate cancer. If your father, brother, or several other blood relatives had prostate cancer, you are more likely to get it as well.

If you have these risk factors, it may be challenging to prevent prostate cancer, but screening frequently and early can help make sure that if you do get cancer, is addressed as soon as possible after being identified.

Diet and lifestyle changes are things you can make.

Prostate cancer is substantially more common among males in western countries than among men in Asia. No one has a conclusive explanation for this occurrence, although specialists believe that variations in eastern and western diets are to blame. Unhealthy eating patterns and diets high in animal proteins and fats can harm DNA and result in cancer.

Men of all ages, ethnicities, and genetic backgrounds can reduce their risk of developing prostate cancer by adopting healthy diets and lifestyles.

1. Make dietary changes

Although studies suggest specific eating habits may be helpful, researchers still don't fully grasp the connection between nutrition and preventing prostate cancer.

• **Consume fewer fats.** Consume fewer saturated and trans fats. • Consume more fruits and vegetables.

• **Emphasize healthy fats, such as omega-3 fatty acids** from fish, nuts, and seeds. Include a wide range of food, especially lots of leafy greens. According to research, the antioxidant lycopene, which is abundant in cooked or processed tomatoes, slows the development of prostate cancer cells. In cruciferous vegetables like broccoli and cauliflower, a compound called sulforaphane is present that may have anti-cancer effects.

• **Add soy and green tea.** Soy may lower PSA levels, and green tea may assist men who are at high risk for prostate cancer reduce that risk, according to clinical trials.

• **Avoid eating burnt meat.** High-temperature charred meat from frying or grilling may develop a chemical component that causes cancer.

2. Keep an Ideal Weight

Prostate cancer can become more aggressive when a person is obese. In general, decreasing weight and keeping it off as you become older will help lower your risk of cancer and numerous other health issues.

3. Workout regularly

Exercise helps battle some of the negative health impacts of a sedentary lifestyle, lower inflammation, and boosts immunological function in addition to assisting you in achieving a healthy weight—all of which can help prevent cancer.

4. Quit smoking and consume less alcohol

One advantage of giving up smoking is a decreased risk of cancer. If you do drink, exercise moderation. According to research, red wine offers antioxidant qualities that may be good for your health.

5. Boost Your Vitamin D Levels

Vitamin D intake is typically inadequate. It can aid in preventing many different illnesses, including prostate cancer. Cod liver oil, wild

salmon, and dried shitake mushrooms are some foods high in vitamin D. Many experts advise receiving 10 minutes of daily sun exposure (without sunscreen) because it is a better and more accessible source of vitamin D. Many doctors recommend vitamin D supplements. However, before taking any vitamin or supplement, see your doctor.

6. Maintain Sexual Activity

According to two studies, men who ejaculate more frequently (with or without a sexual partner) are up to two-thirds less likely to be given a prostate cancer diagnosis. Although research is still being done, some experts believe that ejaculation helps the body get rid of toxins and other things that may otherwise cause inflammation.

Prostate cancer prevention medications

Drugs named finasteride or dutasteride that reduce dihydrotestosterone (DHT) are frequently

used to treat men with benign prostatic hyperplasia (BPH). The effectiveness of these medications in preventing prostate cancer has been thoroughly investigated, and the findings point to a potential 25 percent cancer risk reduction. Discuss the benefits and drawbacks with your doctor because patients who have cancer while taking the medication are more likely to have an aggressive form of the disease.

Natural Methods for Preventing Prostate Cancer

Although there isn't a single natural strategy that works best for everyone, it can help. They include consuming enough fruits and vegetables, exercising, and keeping a healthy weight.

Prostate cancer cannot be prevented, however, it is feasible to lower a person's risk.

If a person follows a doctor's recommendations and exhibits no adverse reaction, the majority of natural means of lowering this risk are safe.

According to research, the following organic compounds may help prevent prostate cancer in some cases:

1. Lycopene

Several studies suggest that regularly consuming lycopene, an antioxidant present in foods like tomatoes and watermelons, may help lower the chance of developing prostate cancer. Nevertheless, there is no evidence to support the

claim that consuming lycopene supplements can lessen the risk of prostate cancer.

2. Calcium D

Many studies have suggested that maintaining high vitamin D levels may help to avoid prostate cancer. Several medical professionals advise increasing your vitamin D levels by taking a daily supplement because it can be difficult to get enough vitamin D only through food sources and sunlight exposure.

3. Omega-3 Fatty Acids

Higher dietary consumption of omega-3 fatty acids was linked to a lower incidence of aggressive prostate cancer, according to a 2009 study involving 466 men with aggressive prostate cancer and 478 age-matched men without prostate cancer. Omega-3s, which are present in oily fish like salmon and mackerel and may help combat prostate cancer by lowering inflammation, according to the study's authors. Other sources are walnuts, flax seeds, and soybeans.

4. Green Tea

Researchers examined information on 49,920 males (aged 40 to 69) for a population study that was published in 2008, and they discovered a connection between drinking green tea and a lower incidence of advanced prostate cancer.

What to Avoid

Certain food additives may make a person more likely to have prostate cancer.
Think twice before avoiding these things
1. Vitamin E and selenium

Selenium and vitamin E were originally thought to be cancer-fighting nutrients by the medical profession.

However, more recent evidence indicates that these substances may raise the risk of prostate cancer in certain persons, whether they are taken together or separately.

Vitamin E and selenium-containing supplements should not be taken by anyone concerned about prostate cancer.

2. Vegetable oils

Several types of cancer are more likely to develop in people who consume excessive amounts of fat, and omega-6 fatty acids found in vegetable oils may encourage the development of prostate cancer cells.

For instance, oils made from corn, sunflower, safflower, cottonseed, and soybeans might have a high omega-6 fatty acid content.

fried or grilled meats

3. Meats cooked at high temperatures, often through grilling or frying, are discouraged by

the National Cancer Institute in the United States.

Muscle meat, such as beef, pork, and chicken, may generate chemicals when cooked at high temperatures, which might alter DNA and raise the chance of developing cancer.

4. carbs and sugar

The glycemic load and glycemic index measurements demonstrate how rapidly sugars and carbs impact a person's insulin and blood sugar levels.

A high glycemic diet may raise the chance of getting prostate cancer, according to certain research.

According to the Dana-Farber Cancer Center, although the link between sugar and cancer is still unclear, these three cancers may be most affected by sugar: pancreatic, prostate, and colorectal.

Other Ways to Avoid Prostate Cancer

Prostate cancer preventive measures might also include eating a diet high in fruits and vegetables, keeping your alcohol consumption to two or fewer drinks per day, exercising for at least 30 minutes each day, and contacting your doctor frequently to have your prostate health monitored.

Make careful to speak with your doctor about the potential advantages and drawbacks of using any kind of dietary supplement for prostate cancer prevention. Self-treatment as well as

putting off or postponing professional medical
care might have detrimental effects.

Conclusion

Prostate cancer is frequently quite treatable
when caught early and given the right care.
Many patients who receive a diagnosis when
cancer has not gone past the prostate continue to
lead healthy lives after therapy for several years.
Yet, in a tiny percentage of cases, the illness can
be aggressive and swiftly spread to other body
parts. Based on your risk factors, your healthcare
professional can talk about the ideal screening
schedule. Depending on how quickly or slowly
your cancer is spreading, they can suggest the
best course of action.

Although prostate cancer cannot be prevented,
certain lifestyle modifications and natural
substances may lower a person's risk.

Attending routine checks and screenings is advised for anyone worried about their chance of developing prostate cancer.

www.ingramcontent.com/pod-product-compliance
Lightning Source LLC
Chambersburg PA
CBHW050801250726
48653CB00030B/2848